YEA[RN]

FOR A CHILD

How to Deal with The Psychological
Effects of Infertility and IVF

Clara Meierdierks
Nee Uwazie

Contribution, Editing and Layout by Amina Chitembo. www.aminachitembo.com
Cover Art by Vivian Timothy.
Cover Designed by Ahsan Chuhadry.
Published by Diverse Cultures Publishing, UK.
Website: www.diverse-cultures.co.uk
Email: publishing@diverse-cultures.co.uk

ISBN: 978-1-9160114-2-7

DEDICATION

I am dedicating this book to the many who have faced the dilemma, stigma and pains of Invitro Fertilisation, and those who are childless for today, tomorrow and in future.

"I have chosen to be authentic, to use my story to teach and empower others, and to learn, as well as to use it to heal my past."

Message of Support and Sincere Respect for My Wife
By Hagen Meierdierks

When the light of my hope, my wife, dazzled me for the first time, I saw a beam of light that was so strong that I simply could not place this unruly power. I only felt as if a voice from the light was calling to me, if not commanding.

Follow Her and Do Not Turn Back. We got to know each other and filtered countless similarities, experiences and parallel out of negative ways of life. The later are stations where you can break, if not break.

One thing, however, has always guided and guided me and my wife the author of this book;

The Belief. It is faith in itself that feeds hope, makes a light visible at the end of the tunnel, and overcomes the stones in the way

The apparently hopeless suffering as described by my wife, the author, in the book, facts could not be richer.

Whether in Nigeria the home country of my wife with all the difficulties and sacrifices you have to deal with and give in order to get ahead or in Germany with all its barricades and pitfalls when you come from a different culture. Relationships that lead to obstruction and collapse.

So, the time comes when that develops, what has evolved from it, namely, that the light leads one to what one is destined and called.

My wife and I have made what we are today out of all our influences in our lives. We are a DOUBLE power in life that fends off all attacks like a wall.

I hope that all those who internalise this book find their own weights and can make life-fulfilling for themselves.

One thing I would like to say to my wife;
I LOVE YOU NKEM.

Visit Clara's Website to Learn More
and check out the latest releases
at: **www.claram.net.**

CONTENTS

INTRODUCTION

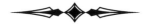

"When you finally gain the courage to share a part of your journey or something that is so private with others, then you realise anyway. It helped put a smile on someone's face, or brightens and revive someone's hopes; it is not only good, but it is also very interesting and beautiful".

- Clara Meierdierks

As Vince Lombardi, an American football coach said; *"The real glory is being knocked to your knees and then coming back. That's real glory. That's the essence of it." Yes, when you go down, family is always the only glory that is left for you.*

Family is considered a strong foundation for a continued strong world. We are in a diversified world and share with different cultures that have different reasons for having children. In the past, in a typical African family, way back where no social system existed. Having many children was considered as a sign of wealth. Children were seen as a great help in farming and were seen as a way of continuity. Families hoped and prayed for more boys as these were seen as the pride to families because they carried on the name of the family, as the girls got married and took the names of their husbands. That link would be lost if a family only had girls, such was the belief in most African cultures. Unfortunately, even till date, Women suffered that pressure to give birth to a boy, and are scorned and abhorred let alone for not having a child at all. This was viewed as an even bigger problem.

Indeed, everyone carries with them some kind of customs and beliefs, this is good and at the same time could hold us sometimes in bondage, it could also serve as a guide to ways of life.

You can imagine what happens to childless African couples and even those that have only one or two children or even only girls. In the Western world, the attitude is quite different, people mind their business, and this takes away a lot of pressure off the couples in the western world, to do their things. Some Arab countries have similar attitude with African belief in dealing with infertility.

When Kate Chopin in her brief novel (Chopin, 1984) The Awakening, Mademoiselle Reiz tells Edna, "The bird that would soar above the level of plain tradition and prejudice must have strong wings, she did not make any mistake, she was right. It is still a sad spectacle to see the weaklings bruised, childless couple exhausted, frustrated and suffered when things go contrary to societal expectations.

However, the aim of this book is to help couples yearning for a child to be well informed about the psychological effects of infertility and the IVF journey(HFEA, 2019; NHS, 2019), and to give them some tools to deal with the ups and downs they may encounter in the process, based on my personal experience. It is also to encourage them not to give up hopes even when the journey is accompanied with failure and disappointment, because it is only those who persevere and never give up that succeed.

The book **'Yearning for a Child'** stems from my personal experience as an insider, who has known the ups and downs that goes with not having a child for years. Moreso,` The ride of yearning for a child `is perceived differently in many cultures, for example, in African culture where I come from. Infertility comes with insurmountable pressure of constant questioning and nagging from families and society and from those who know when one got married.

In most cases, women are blamed for infertility and are given all sorts of titles and names for not having children. A woman who has no children can be considered as having done something wrong in the past, and this is viewed in some cultures as some kind of a curse or punishment. Some in-laws can be extremely unforgiving to a woman who is not bringing a child to the family. The blame is the same whether the problem is with the man or from the woman, the woman tends to suffer the most.

In any case, childlessness in the context of today may be ´willingly or not Willingly desired, for an African, childlessness is not a choice rather is considered by the society as a problem. We are in a diversified world, and It is my hope that those reading this book will be encouraged and equipped to deal with the psychological stress, stigma and pains that goes with this journey.

To give the most benefit of this book; I start by explaining Infertility, Invitro Fertilisation IVF, and Intracytoplasmic Sperm Injection (ICSI) (Mastenbroek et al., 2011) in which case a healthy single sperm is injected into a mature egg under a very strict sterile environment. This is done in cases where the problem of infertility is caused by the male partner in the simplest form. I will also explain some of the ways in which some African cultures look at these high techs today and some ways of dealing with the psychological stress that goes with infertility and IVF based on personal experience and encounter with some couples I met in the process of my journey. I had the privilege of interviewing two different couples who had had a similar experience. Having listened to the agonies of some other people who are of Immigrant background, I decided I should write this book to let many in this pain know that they are not alone in this journey.

Infertility: remain one of the reasons for broken marriages in African context of today. However, the truth is that every woman can be a good mother, even when it is not your biological child, but people need to get rid of this myth . There are so many ways of achieving motherhood. Unfortunately, people are blinded by societal definitions of infertility and encapsulate in this belief.

Sadly, most of us shy away from discussing 'infertility' let alone our personal experiences, adoption or even surrogacy is a taboo topic, this is either due to some cultural beliefs, our mentality, and societal definition of all these. Yes, there are so far some articles that have dealt with some influence of social and cultural factors on infertility and new reproductive technologies and our interpretations of them. For example, people of African background are worst tortured psychologically when pregnancy fails to take place as dictated by the society in which one finds himself, unfortunately, this class of people, rather die in silence than openly discussing infertility problems. There is indeed a need for sharing personal journey on this topic to increase awareness in different context that has failed to understand the word infertility. Unfortunately, not many of this information gets to the people concerned.

Frank Van Balen, researched on such topics like childlessness, reasons for having children and families in which he states that some parenthood came from the use of a new reproductive technology called IVF (Invitro Fertilisation) termed today as medical wonder. Unfortunately, there is indeed a strong relationship to our perception of childlessness, IVF, adoption, surrogacy and culture.

Moreover, where one is born, determines how these issues are addressed and perceived.

In any case, It is very necessary to read wide and think not only on the horizon of culture and people around but rather to think beyond the natural ways of being pregnant and having children. Thank God that today the route to parenthood has been widened and thank God who put knowledge in researchers of Anthropology of Reproduction, sociology, ethics, Public health, and women's studies. The world is different and changing, so one's attitude and perceptions about all these should also change.

New technology as reported by Henry M.W, Bos and Floor B, Van Rooij 2009 has resulted in more than 300,000 babies since its discovery. In the past infertility was only seen as a fault that needed only medical intervention, even when it fails to work, couples were not seriously given attention, because some culture stigmatised it and defined INFERTILITY to suit their terms and conditions. In Africa, even till today, child-less couples, especially women are considered to have done something grave in their youth days that affected their inability to become pregnant, such are our beliefs.

Thank God, there is hope to deal with this issue. There is hope for the many who have lost hope, hope to begin again, and ply the many routes to a dream. My background as an African puts a lot of importance on having children, hence, this book is to increase the hopes of women who would ordinarily go under culture and people's judgements, and also to encourage many in this, to embrace and accept the new technology that enhances pregnancy when natural ways fail us, don't mind those side talks. there is nothing to be ashamed of.

Moreover, most of us should be assured that IVF is not a taboo and not a crime. It is just like any other pregnancy. The fact that it did not happen naturally as defined by society, and just that it is seen as medically or surgically assisted using a high technology does not make it any different, after all, people take some kind of drugs to enable or enhance their chances of being pregnant, some even take local herbs to get pregnant.

So why are people being secretive about IVF? And why won't people explore other options if they desperately want `Maternal bliss.` ?.

I aim to be open with this topic, so that I can help as many people as possible. When you are open, you will quickly realise that people will not be curious and somewhat nosy about your situation because you have pre-empted their gossip.

I have written more about my journey through IVF in my chapter in The Perfect Migrant book and my first solo book "The Long Struggle to Discovering Me." In the two books, I discussed a lot about what my IVF journey was like. I must confess that after so many years of inside work within and outside me, and after a long deliberation on my psychological ride of yearning for a child and getting blessed after many failed efforts.

Having encountered with people who have had failed IVFs, some good people around me and some testimonies from people like Celine Dion and her late husband Rene sharing their IVF journey on YouTube, and many others in this quest for motherhood, I was indeed encouraged to do something . I said wow, I am not doing what someone has not done before. CelineDion and her husband also went through six attempts like I did and they were not ashamed to talk about it. For me, I am sharing my experience to pass on the baton. I hope to share this story in full. As this is a story of pain and ultimate joy, to help others in this ride to tap into my story and get going.

I struggled and am still struggling within me on whether this story will get to the target and focus audience. I did not initially feel good about sharing my journey. I do not know about what others think. Still I believe these are some doubts we go through when we want to share our personal journeys. I am especially dedicating this book to those who are still in this struggle and quest for *"Maternal bliss"* for today, tomorrow and in future.

You can never find the right answers to a lot of things; however, you can gain inspiration reading other people's stories, especially from ordinary people who have gone through the ride before you. Don't limit yourself, don't see yourself through the eyes of others; they are not the ones to define you.

When it gets too much,
Spare your energy,
Cry to God,
Because He is not a God that has no feelings,
So, pray even when you are happy,
He will hear you.

We all have something, stories, experiences, or journeys that have failed us. We sometimes choose not to talk about them. Well, it is a personal decision.

I have chosen to be authentic, to use my story to teach and empower others and to learn, as well as to use it to heal my past.

As the mighty Bruce Lee once said; If you follow the classical pattern, you are understanding the routine, the tradition, the shadow, you are not understanding yourself. So understanding oneself and being oneself is truly an act that needs to be mastered by many who wishes to be happy in their situation.

WHAT A JOURNEY.

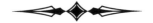

When we allow Life to guide us, and we decide to step into the process with a positive mindset, not forgetting that daring fear gives us the strength to decide our future, we will accomplish a lot instead of being in the way of our future. We all make mistakes, but, we should not forget that mistakes are there to serve a reference and guide. When we fall we feel the Pains, and it is this pains that remind us that we are still alive and on a journey and being alive tells us that we have not lost, that victory can still be achieved, if we fight harder, struggle harder and persevere unceasingly, we will not only dream dreams, we would be able to realise our set dreams.

The Sun Will Definitely Shine for You

Don't forget no road is without thorns.
So take up your fate, and accomplish your goal,
No dream comes easy.
So don't sit down and get drown in your past mistakes.
As for our dreams,
Never were good goals achieved without pains,
Yes !we 'll go through,
The agonies that go with our dreams.
The stumbling, the personal fights,
And the inner doubts of; can we, why not this and that?
There will be loss of courage,
Wars within self,
And the desire to give up.

Tears will be shed, but tears alone.
Will not heal the wounds incurred.
And make good the troubled heart.

You will hear things,
Things that may sicken you.
Moments that will make you feel rejected,
And hate yourself,
Yes, a trying moment indeed.
For those in this journey.

If you are one in this kind of ride,
A kind of ride that shaken faith, croaks and
entangles,
That Robs and steals sleep.
When it grips,
It knows no pity
When it grips,
* It let loose a heavy force*
That press your whole being,
And make you powerless,

It may take a cruel hold on your mental health,
And may become your jungle test,
surfacing with trials and failures.
That blurs and disjoints reasonings,

Yes, you could be so clouded with
Grief, but don't be lost,
Cry but hold your head,
Get lost but find yourself

Embrace the adversity,
Endure, Pray, be positive, and be persistent.

Put your feet down,
Print success in mind,
Follow your heart,
and not their judgements,
for they will let your hopes down,
never mind, they will talk,
But do yourself a favour,
Fight your fight,
Follow your dreams,
And print your success,

Yes!
Persevere, pray and hold, hold and hold on to
HIM,
For Tomorrow and one day
The sun will definitely shine for you.

Many of us will not have gone through this lane before, and many will need to be very persistent like Hannah in 1 Kings in the Holy Bible. Hannah was reported as being barren; she was many times provoked by her rival, yes, so is the case with some in this ride for a child. Hannah in the Bible suffered barrenness for years. She would cry and refuse to neither sleep nor eat and could not be consoled until she started getting answers from above. Yes, although the priest in the church mistook her persistent cry for being drunk, no she was not, she was not drunk, she needed answer, and she got her Solomon from God.

One lesson she taught us was unceasingly honestly asking for God´s intervention through prayers for those who believe in God, persistence, and perseverance helps in any difficult situation.

People like Eli, the priest thought she was drunk; she wasn't drunk; she was yearning for a child, just like any other woman in need. Hannah, like many, suffered some psychological pains from other women and from society. Hannah was quick to understand that God hears cries. She cried her eyeballs out, as she carried all to God. She asked God several questions and kept sleepless nights just like any other woman yearning for a child. Hannah Knew the joy of having a child, and knew what to do, as she was never meant to give up her dreams. In the end, God made her dream come through.

What happened in the end?

God gave her Samuel, a son that wiped her tears and fulfilled her yearnings for a child. Yes, it was not IVF, but her persistence, hope, and unceasing prayers gave answers to her worries.

Anyway, our stories may not end like Hannah's case, but we could borrow her kind of faith and fight our various challenges like her. In life we all may not be a winner, We win sometimes and lose also, but in any case, we should not completely lose our orientation, our target, and our dreams, because when we lose focus, we live to regret. I honestly, don't wish anyone to go through this IVF ride, but if it is the only option left. Tears, prayers, good network, and a healthy environment are necessary for this journey.

The Unpredictable.

"Navigating the unexpected in one's life requires great emotional courage- the courage to be nothing and nobody for a while as you question who you have and who you want to be."

- Barbara de Angelis.

Understanding the complexity of this journey is seen as one way of moving forward, and one way of understanding who you are.

I never knew this could happen to anyone until I found myself in this ride. I was living a quiet life full of struggles, and never thought of such a huge challenge, until I became a nobody who questioned `who I am `and `What I want to be!

Yes! Who do I want to be? In the face of IVF challenges! A fighter, a runaway, a believer and or strong woman.

For me to live my dreams, meant going through a tough journey and not doing anything half way.

It was not easy though, but became very necessary for me to bear in mind that failures, and doubts, unpredictability makes up parts of this journey, but in the face of all these challenges, God the almighty was always my guide and made a way for me . When we believe, and do the right things, God´s light will surely shine for us, no matter how long.. However, Prayers, perseverance, and getting the right mindset have yielded a great success story in dealing with Infertility issues, as testified by many who have faced this challenge in the past.

You may be lucky and have your IVF success in one attempt. But if you happen to find yourself in many trips, I suggest you begin putting things down in paper, because, it might be a weapon to tell your story in future.

IVF RIDE
Rough, difficult as it may be,
With its unpredictability,
And doubts, Fears, pain aches,
That Clouds and shadow the mind,
Doubts that envelop the mind,
And choke up reasoning,
And multiply misery,
This damn hold when it set
 discomforts and depresses,
And will spare you not.
Whatever the feelings, the obstacles you
Encounter in your own journey,
Embrace your pain,
Turn it to your strength, and;
Your journey will be yours,"

It is always our wish to end any journey well. Unfortunately, having all information concerning a journey does not always mean that the journey will end up well, when it does we are so grateful to God, and when it turns out the other way round, we become sad, disappointed and even get discouraged, this is human and is not forbidden, so feel free and don't be hard on yourself when the going gets tough.

What Is this Journey About?

"Permanence, perseverance, and persistence in spite of all obstacles, discouragements and impossibilities: It is this, that in all things, distinguishes the strong from the weak"

-Thomas Carlyle.

Yes if you succeed in the end, you are strong and not weak,

You are bold and have faith,

Yes, this will distinguish you truly,

This is a journey of a struggle to have a baby through IVF. It is a real challenge, a hard journey. I must confess, and not a bed of roses. So be prepared to take up whatever challenges it has to offer you, as a woman.

Who Is A Woman?

A woman is defined biblically in Genesis 2:18-25 as bone and flesh of a man, and this is why a man leaves his father and mother and becomes attached to his wife, and they become one flesh.

Yes the woman houses, nurtures, and labour.

See the artwork of my sister Vivian Timothy, the beautiful painting of a mother with her child on her back, no cover would have being more suitable to speak the joy of a family.

Oh! That is a woman, She is strong, multi-tasking, a mother a wife and everything. Yes, she is a woman with organs that naturally is meant for forming and carrying pregnancy for 9months, yes that is a Woman carrying a baby on her back with pride,a woman with love and passion. Oh! Yes oo, she is a woman with more to offer....

For the sake of understanding the process, this book will make a bit of explanation about the reproductive system of a woman in the simplest way possible, because knowing and understanding our reproductive system is very vital to planning a family.

However everyone should know her body, hence I am including a little information to this effect. The female reproductive organ includes the uterus, the Fallopian tubes and Ovaries. I have derived the definitions from the book 'A

General Textbook of Nursing' (Pearce, 1980), in order to clarify things to my readers.

THE UTERUS is believed to be a hollow organ, shaped like a flattened pear and is situated in the middle of the true pelvis. Said to be divided into 3 parts, the Fundus, Body, and Isthmus that connect to the Cervix, with its significant functions; this is accordingly about 7.5cm long, 5cm wide and 2.5cm deep and weighs 65g. The uterus is said to have a very good blood supply and lymphatic drainage.

THE CERVIX is a canal with the internal and external mouth. It is a link to the Vagina and the Uterus. Very important during labour process.

THE UTERINE WALL is an Endometrium the inner lining that has high hormonal control from puberty to cessation of blood.

THE MYOMETRIUM is kind of muscular in layers and forms the thickness of the uterine wall. It plays a great role in pregnancy and delivery.

THE PERIMETRIUM is another kind of layer, said to cover the surface of the uterus.

THE FALLOPIAN TUBES are said to be about 10cm long, muscular. They are found on either side of the uterus, extending to the pelvis, with each attached either side of the uterus. It is very close to the ovary and plays a great role in Menstruation and pregnancy. There are layers, with each tube having four parts, the interstitial, isthmus and ampulla a stretch out portion, and the infundibulum with its finger-like, that serve to catch up with the fertilised egg and aid the transport back to the uterus for transplantation it aids the transport to and fro of sperm and the return of the fertilised eggs back to their normal position. The uterus serves for implantation and growth of a baby.

THE OVARIES are Described in the general textbook of nursing from Evelyn Pearce as two Almond shaped organs situated inside a peritoneal cavity, posterior to the fallopian tubes. Each said to consists of inner medulla, outer cortex.

The ovaries are responsible for the production of ova, or eggs for fertilisation, and the production of hormones to aid implantation and maintain pregnancy when it occurs for the first three months and if no pregnancy, this follows the menstrual cycle with the preparation of the endometrium for likely pregnancy occurrence and menstruation or shedding of endometrial lining of the uterus.

First day of the menstrual period to the first of the next constitutes menstrual cycle, although duration of cycle varies, 28 days is said to be common cycle.

This is what happens at puberty, the anterior lobe of the pituitary gland produces two Gonadotrophic sex-gland stimulating hormones, to enhance the work of ovarian follicles.

OVULATION according to Evelyn Pearce, occurs 14 days prior to next menstruation. As girls mature in life, this follows ripening of Follicles that produces oestrogen and release of eggs called Ovum at the rupture of the follicles when it ripens, it is slimy and breaks out when riped as it is attracted and drawn to end of fallopian tube to be transported into the uterine cavity, which when semen is present leads to union of egg and ova resulting to fertilisation .

Follicle stimulating hormone (FSH) this controls the ripening of the Graafian follicle in the ovary, the production of Oestrogen and the discharge of the ripened ovum. The ripening of the Graafian follicle, increases in size, becomes transparent, projects from the surface of the ovary, ruptures and is swept away with the help of the follicular fluids, then trapped by the end of the fallopian tube and transported into the uterine cavity. This occurs 14 days prior to the beginning of the next menstrual cycle.

The Luteinising hormone (LH) is said to stimulate the growth of the corpus luteum where the Graafian follicles have ruptured. This produces progesterone that gets the endometrium lining ready for reception of ovum, which if no fertilisation, the corpus luteum disintegrates after 12days, production of progesterone reduces, causing the endometrial lining to break down and sheds its lining in form of menstruation.

FERTILISATION takes place in the fallopian tube(Finger like), as semen reaches the tube through its swimming actions, this then pierces the egg, and fertilise it by uniting with the semen, cell division of the fertilised egg follows.

This, in turn, passes through the tube(s) and back to the uterine cavity for implantation. Following this, changes occur in the woman, more oestrogen and progesterone are produced, to maintain the pregnancy.

PREGNANCY follows with early symptoms of morning sickness around 6 - 7 weeks. The breast changes at 4 weeks due to oestrogen and progesterone effect. Abdominal fullness and eventual increase in the uterus size, between 8 and 20 weeks, a lot of changes would have taken place. Many clinics and gynaecologists now recommend pregnancy test from the 9 -14 days of missing a period, to ascertain pregnancy.

Some test like HCG Immunological tests for detecting human Chorionic gonadotrophin are new inventions and are some of the medical wonders used to detect early pregnancy.

This is what happens when it all goes well for a couple. God willing in 40 weeks from the start of the process, they will have their pride and joy. The baby or babies. Unfortunately, things do not always go according to plan and some pregnancies fail.

WHAT HAPPENS WHEN PREGNANCY FAILS TO OCCUR NATURALLY? WHO GETS THE BLAME?

When couples stay together for six months or more and no pregnancy occurs naturally, if not planned. Anxiety sets in and those around begin to count dates. Sometimes it is the external pressure from the people around that causes most of the anxiety. The next thing, the couple becomes unconsciously uncomfortable as worry sets in.

The woman checks her pants every month, each time she sees her monthly bleeding after many months of staying with her husband, she becomes so unhappy, and makes moves to see a gynaecologist who after series of test may confirm `Infertility` which could either be her fault or that of her husband.

WHAT IS INFERTILITY AND WHAT DOES IT MEAN IN OUR CONTEXT?

How infertility is perceived has a lot to do with our culture and religion. For example, the way and manner in which the affected couples are watched and monitored in African communities and in Africa is different compared to developed countries, where people mind their business.

Africans especially, have a compound way of life where one's problem is viewed as everyone´s problem. Even when you think it is your life, no, cultural beliefs of an average African make women vulnerable to blame. An African woman must be a mother, otherwise…

A CHILDLESS WOMAN IN AFRICA

Cries and rattles within, thinking, murmuring, crying and staying awake all the nights,

Asking, wondering, seeking answers and wonder-
ing why,
Pondering, figuring on the mystic of her womb,
Mother nature she questions,
 pleading, asking why me!
 Why, why, she is thorned,
woed, denied and pitied,
From normal woman barred sanctioned
And isolated,
Cursed and ill-treated,
For nature's denial of her maternal bliss,

please, I plead! Don't touch her,
Please don't make her feel empty,
Please don't be the cause of her many tears,
Save her from more agony,
Give her love,
 she is still human, with feelings,
Human-like you despite infertility,
Strong, enterprising and good-hearted,
Please don't say she is the reason,
She is loving, caring, and a woman,

Only denied a child by nature.
Yes, she is a woman without a child,
Who Stands and wonder in her head.
Would I ever be a mother?

Would I ever suckle children?
Would I….. with the weights choking her,

She is a woman a normal woman,
She gets the pains,
the blames and all the bad fingers.
Abhorred by culture,
Defined and stigmatized,
Yes, she is a woman that wants to be a mother
But could not,
It is not her choice
So don,t speak into her ears,
Don't whisper behind her
and mock her in her face,

Mother-in-law call her good name,
Show her empathy,
She did not choose to be childless,

Don't chase her out of her marriage,
Don't walk her away and ask her to leave your son.
Don't be a reason for her tears and her keeping awake at night,

She has cried enough, and her eyeballs are bulging,
She bid to find answers,

From God ! and not you,

Yes ! the questions and torment goes on,
Until she breaks or leaves or finds answers,
A broken African woman.
Lonely without a child!
Yes! the agony of an African childless woman.

Unfortunately, women suffer more when pregnancy fails to occur naturally in an African context. She is called names and even accused of living wayward life in her young years. In extreme cases when perhaps, with years gone by with no positive results seen, the in-laws could be the one to force the woman out of her marital home.

If you happen to have a horrible mother-in-law or sisters-in-law they could even accuse you of being a man.

Read this interview from Mr and Mrs. Q perhaps you will understand the agony of some childless African women.

I have decided not to disclose the names for the sake of privacy. Here it goes:

ME: Good morning! mmmm

I stammered to the couple, while focusing more on the lady, who was looking so downcast, and so sad. It took me a while before I was able to go to this couple, inside I prayed so that they will not think I am not mindful of my business.

Behold, I found out that they needed someone to cry unto, A shoulder to lean on and let their woes out. I gave them that:

An ear that could listen
while they talk and talk,
without interruption.
I listened to their words
And I attended to them
And my words were shaped from my experience,
The things that I have gone through,
Gave me wisdom.

In all sincerity, I spoke to them. As I urged them to take up their fights, their challenges and channel to God. I know when we do the right thing. We must let God in. He will do the fight for us. He will send a mediator. He will send a messenger to remind us that it is not finished.

Listen to me I said to them,
What it was like with me.
May I ask why you are looking so sad, I proceeded
with my question.

Mrs Q: busted out in tears, for one hour, she wept uncontrollably, like a child.
ME: Please can I hug you, I said to her,
Mrs Q: did not hesitate to wrap her arms around me.

AT A QUIET CORNER: After a while, I introduced myself, meanwhile this encounter happened years back, at my 4th IVF attempt at UNI ESSEN, GERMANY.
MR. Q: Was also looking so worried, as I noticed the anxious looks I made eye contact with Mrs Q, as I held her hand. In order to calm them down, I decided to tell them a bit of my ordeal so as to gain their trust and at the same time, let them know that they were not alone.

I am a woman who suffered separation with a previous relationship; I started off with my story. I Suffered and got shut off from call it maternal bliss, nature or luck, with no hope of establishing a new beginning before my biological clock started to ring bell.
It was as if my dreams were never to be realised. I wept inside and outside during the period of the previous relationship. There were no obvious

problems with me, at least all medical checks, no Dr. could say there was anything wrong with me. I never ever thought my life could go through this, as it dawned on me that my partner then had a problem, I finally accepted to walk the lane, each time I sigh heavily, Oh! Was I not going to carry a baby?

For me, I was bereaved, that was just how I felt at the thought of everything. I did not have any act of mastering this pain,

I suffered from personal rejection by me, and I refused to accept what was happening.

I never ever identified with the situation, at first, Still, I did not let go my dreams,

Rather I choose to Seek for answers and never wanted to give up.

I looked around and wondered If Motherhood has slipped away from me,

Dominating my thoughts were why me!

I wondered If I ever will be a mom of a child, children? A teacher and everything to a child.

The more I thought of this, the more depressed I became,

I felt so shut out, so lost and rejected,

I could not give me that kind of support I needed,
let alone the society,
Where am I going to go for answers,
Who will wipe my tears!
Were my many worries,

For the first time in this journey, my fate was seriously shaken,
But my hunger for a baby never stopped,

Lo! Seeking out, for reassurance and answers, sidelined my Thought, but still, I remained strong enough to pursue and never gave my dreams up.

Having listened to a part of my story, the lady threw her arms around me again and began to sob for a while, in the end we all left tapping strength from our experiences so far.

You don't want to imagine what Mrs. Q told me about her ordeal. If you are of African origin, the rest you can figure out yourself.

A childless African woman is bound to suffer societal pressure; they are excluded and are lonely. They are gradually dropped out and forgotten as well as even mocked. Even when you find yourself in the midst of other parents, discussions are usually centred mostly on their children, which could be quiet painful to a woman who never chose to be childless.

Can you tell a childless African couple not to worry to become a mother or to experience motherhood, this is not in line with Africa, because in African context children mean wealth, protection, continuation and others, now you see why African context are unable to accommodate any woman without a child whether biological or adopted . Thank God, in this 21st century, there are lots of many other ways one can quench the yearn for a child. Just seek out for information.

Incidentally, the couple referred here were Nigerians, from Ibo land, it was just coincidence that brought us together and made us exchange experience. Wow, you can't imagine how helpful it feels sharing your story, especially with those in the same journey. Nonetheless, I found myself at that moment to be stronger, despite my own pains then. Such is the agony of an African couple looking for maternal bliss.

THE INFERTILITY SAGA

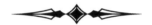

Imagine when different doctors tell you that there was nothing wrong with you, still every month you keep on having this menstrual ache, warning you for a monthly period. This becomes annoying as hunger for being a mom increases. This put huge strain on my previous relationship. At 35, my hopes were still very high, with 43 my previous relationship broke up, and I feared I would never be a mother.

I planned writing this book on this topic for a long time, to encourage women still having the hopes of being biological moms. Often, childless women are not treated well by society that should protect them. I am investing energy in this writing to encourage childless moms to feel good and seek out for other options, for one could still be a good mom without being a biological mom.

However, Infertility and highlighted on what is normal infertility. Reportedly, about 85% of couple in the study were said to have achieved natural pregnancy in one year, 7% reportedly in two years. To this effect, infertility has come to be defined as an inability to conceive within 12 months of marriage or being in partnership obgyn.ucla.edu.

The American Pregnancy association (American Pregnancy Association, 2019) say on their website that:

> "infertility is a condition that affects approximately 1 out of every 6 couples. An infertility diagnosis is given to a couple that has been unsuccessful in efforts to conceive over the course of one full year. When the cause of infertility exists within the female partner, it is referred to as female

infertility. Female infertility factors contribute to approximately 50% of all infertility cases, and female infertility alone accounts for approximately one-third of all infertility cases. However, these days Couples are advised to seek medical advice when they feel it is not working out."

I tell you, infertility in most African culture starts from the minute a man and woman come together, and if after two months, there were no pregnancy forthcoming, and no exhibition of signs of pregnancy, as is expected from the man's family, the woman is automatically stamped 'INFERTILE'. This is how culture defines all in this course, as the couple face and silently battles their uncertainties.

Uncertainty of Life

"The difference between stumbling blocks and stepping stones is how you use them"

– Unknown.

We go through life process with uncertainties. Maybe is even best to deal with the unknown. At any stage of one's life, is some kind of challenge waiting. For every couple IVF is a kind of a big challenge, and I truly do not even wish any woman to go through this pains, I wish all yearning for children to have a natural journey, if not in IVF journey, when one records a failure of the cycle more than once, it becomes agonising and a stumbling block for other plans, whatever, all that matters is how you go about it.

As for me, It was a huge challenge, a process of life, that needed to be mastered and embraced with faith, hope and perseverance. It is indeed my hope that this book will spur a lot in this journey, to keep going until your dreams come through. To say life was going to be easy, no one can predict. It is very natural to get doubts and get doubted in the process of yearning for a baby, for life has its own laws and regulates its own rules.

We go through troubles sometimes and have our faces hide our worries in smiles. What the heart harbours is often far from what is visible. To get to our destinations, my God, I said silently very often some of us go through pains, go through sleepless nights, worry our heads, and even loose hopes. Nonetheless, I never at any point think for a moment that things could turn out the way they did in the past. Today, when I look back, I murmur within me, 'Me' a mother of a beautiful bundle of joy `!, Glory to God.

The fact is that, somethings in life gets unbearably hard sometimes before it gets going. In whatever bad situation you find yourself, perseverance is the answer,

"For nothing in the world can take the place of persistence. Talent will not; nothing is more common than unsuccessful men with talent. Genius will not; unrewarded genius is almost a proverb. Education will not; the world is full of educated derelicts. Persistence and determination alone are omnipotent. The slogan Press On! has solved and always will solve the problems of the human race."

- Calvin Coolidge.

Yes, I did not stop half way and I did not listen to their judgement, Yes! I pressed on and the Lord saw me through.

WHEN WE THINK

What a joy,
What luck,
We feel when we start off,

When we find love
When we think we find a smile?
A laugh and a partner,

When we Suddenly,
 start feeling compromised,
And uncomfortable,

Hmmmm!
We feel stucked,
Imprisoned and lost,
We realise even hope eludes us in time of challenge,
When our yearn for a child is dashed,
Relationship broken,
We get lost in search,
In yearn for a child,
And in quest for who we are,

Hmmmm!
They will pinch you,
And matters turn strangely,
The mind gets to work,
And dominates with worries
Like many persons in this,

With clouded thoughts!
Can I?

Will I?
Complete my Family?
And be someone's biological mom.

Why Longing For Family

We long for families because of what they stand for. They stick together families are happier by far than the brothers and the sisters who take separate highways, FAMILY ARE :

"The happiest people living, are the wholesome folks who make a circle at the fireside that no power, but death can break."

- Edgar Guest.

Yes family is the only thing only death can break in this physical world. No wonder anyone feels incomplete without family.

Starting a family is very exciting because of what family stands for. It is beautiful but it could sometimes turn out the other way, especially when infertility rovers around, and that is when you need your family most. When it does not work out, please don't destroy yourself, seek help, look out and find those who are in this journey, you are not alone and will never be alone. You are not the first and will not be the last; there are so many in this journey; you only need to search for them to give you the right coping mechanism, but hold on to your family.

Whenever we go down, families that stick together will always win, no matter the weight of the trial, family will be the last to leave.

So many things in life are very uncertain, and that makes it somehow unpredictable in such a journey like IVF. If you have a family that will give you support, you are blessed. I do not intend to dramatize anything to cloud against the moment or dampen your spirit. I have trailed on this path before, not once and not twice, am just one in a million that have gone through this lane, many times. I am writing from the point of an insider, who has known the agony of this journey, the dilemma, stigma, pains and the isolation that goes with it. Above all, the joy of a family.

Despite whatever uncertainty and hardships IVF journey threw in my path, one thing I didn't do was to quit my dream, I held on to my faith, my yearning for a child was stronger than any challenges, even after many storms in my life. I held on to faith, to God, I intensified, because, I know that life and all that happened with us, are just a process of life. I love family ways of doing things, and that is a beautiful thing about family.

We don't choose to fail in any things we decide or choose to do; it could be that things fail us along the way, which is certain to happen at times in this ride. Call it anything, but I prefer to call it a psychological ride.

Let us go back to some facts now. Here are some factors that can delay pregnancy.

- *Unhealthy sperm or no sperm cell (Azoospermia) few sperms called Oligospermia.*
- *Man can also have a genetic deformity of sperm*
- *The strength and motility of the sperm.*
- *Women's unhealthy eggs.*
- *The state of the Fallopian tubes.*
- *Lack of ovulation*
- *Congenital problems*
- Age of the couple especially the woman (hormonal production ability) (Still wonders happen).
- The state of the endometrine wall.
- Quality of the fertilised egg.

As explained to me by all the specialists I encountered, and of course from my knowledge as a nurse and midwife and physiological practitioner.

SOCIETAL
EXPECTATIONS

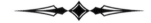

The societal expectations on a couple can sometimes be harsh and unforgiving. We live in a world where people do not mind their business. Everyone gets involved and murmur at your back. This can be counterproductive and hurtful when the couple is going through a challenging period.

We learn to be resilient, despite the pain, learn to pretend, we don't care, until we can simply push ugly thoughts away, because the societal, cultural influence in our lives, help shape who we truly are and how we respond to failures.

When things work out for us,
Joy abounds, and thoughts are good,
They world fill different
And radiate joy.

The same world starts to move,
The minute one comes together,
stay together, the count time,
and thick tack for you,

It is time they tell you,
Time for answers,
Answers to their expectations,

Their eyes want to see
The change and the bulge,
That goes with couples' times together.

They will look out for signs,
Signs of body changing,
They will ask, if it has happened,
And they want to see and see,

When after a while,
Nothing happens,
They will mimic, gossip,
And will give you pains.

Then begins the agony.

One thing common in African context is that
we do not mind our business

After the union of a man and a woman, especially after marriage, pregnancy is expected from the society to follow, when it fails to happen, again and again, worries set in about what people will think.

We all are trapped in our cultural beliefs and the norms that define who we are, what should happen to us at a set of time, and so on. In my case, I was in there before I realised what I was in for.

How often have I read about this?
Thinking of them,
And not me?
O yes,
I defined it for them,
And I prayed words of encouragement
For them,

When I write,
It was for them and not me,
And suddenly,
I too could be them,
And not them,
Yes,
I became one of them,
Yearning for children
Yes, I became

Them that were culturally defined and marginalised.

Yes!
I did not escape the dark side
of this ride.
Here is me,
And not them
Yes, you could be them,

I met a man before my husband and the father of our daughter, and just like any new relationship, all initially looked rosy, and there was never any sign that all was not well.

We tried to get pregnant naturally; however after six months, nothing had happened, as a woman, I got so worried and discussed with him on what could be the possible reasons.

Out of respect for him, I will reserve the details of his comments and reactions. What happened next was to take a bold step to consult a doctor.

The Doubts

"Doubts kill more dreams than failure ever will."

- Suzy Kassem.

Unfortunately, even when one pretends to be strong especially at some stages of IVF journey, doubts accompanies one.

Our doubts our worries,
Our fight, our fears,
We fear, we worry,
We doubt everything,
Including our dreams
As we wonder, Will it?
Yes, will it,
Doubt a companion.

Many will ask if the infertility is the fault of the woman alone. Of course, we are in a patriarchal

world where men are not easily accused of anything that is the world we live in.

The first thing that comes to mind when a
couple is not getting pregnant is `the woman `
people´s first finger will be pointed at the woman
as the reason for delayed pregnancy, yes, the
woman, the weaker being in the eyes of men,it is
`she `who would take the blame.

Research shows that a third of the infertility is related to men's issues, the other one third
to women. The remaining one third relates to
shared problems.

After six months to one year depending on
where you come from, couples are advised to
take the next move. Most shy away and most in
the world of today seek for help.

Reality Sets In

Of course, just like anyone in a relationship,
expectations were mounted and huge on us. I
could say in my mind and plead with the society
not to put too much pressure on me, I would
want to tell them to leave me at my own pace,
but this I can not influence and my partner then,
was the foot mat on which his family tumbles
and step on.

I was so silent about my journey and wanted it so, as I did not let many people know about what I suffered in silence. I expected an easy life, easy slip to motherhood, but all I faced was difficulties, trials and pains that accompany the quest for maternal bliss In my widest dream, I would not have imagined this kind of journey, but yes I did, I went to places, in search of answers. What made the journey so miserable was the then partner and his family. Perhaps, it could not have been that traumatising, if not for the pressures the put on me, both in words and acts.

I went about wearing a mask beneath, a mask that only me can feel and touch, a mask that was invisible to people that covered my pains, and shielded me from the world. I would go out to work, and no one suspected the burden beneath.

The First Visit to a Doctor.

In our case, after the anticipation and worries, it was time to take the next move. The next move meant making an appointment with a gynaecologist, who after series of examinations, said the results seemed okay, however still after nothing was happening. We then had a referral to an infertility clinic for further clarifications, and the first visit landed us at Düsseldorf teaching hospital at the fertility department.

The visit called for the initial experiments, that included taking a general history from both of us.

A series of tests followed by the use of Clomide a tablet that stimulates ovulation. Still, nothing happened; it was then time for the man's checklist tests.

The test on my partner indicated a problem, which is usually supressed and lost in culture, leaving the woman as a figure that should be blamed.

When eventually all were cleared emotional tumult set in, because the next step could mean, another total check of both, as well as psychological, and genetical tests, all these are recommended procedures. They generated pains, worries and doubts.

Things like Hystero salphingogram HSG, dye is injected into the uterine tubes, to check if there is any blockage, as the fallopian tubes have major role to play in one getting pregnant. The role was mentioned earlier on one of the page…

If no blockage of tubes and if no fibroids or growths are detected anywhere, which could be a hindrance if hormone levels are adequate. Any woman is ready at this point to do whatever, even if it means undergoing many surgical operations.

If the test of the man indicates, poor sperm quality, low motility and morbidity, at the end, the doctor tells you both, you will need to try this and that, if in the end, nothing happens, an IVF – is recommended, as it was with my previous relationship- As Dr K called us in to tell us of the many options available: IVF, Surrogacy; Donor; Adoption etc. Guess what followed.

The Dilemma

Feeling Low After the News.
I address my poem to pain,
As I used my pen to eulogise this very pain,
Of all the pains, you are so strong,
Stronger than I imagined,
Harder and heart-breaking,
Cruel and clinging,
Replacing smiles with fear,
in every point

Infertility in Modern Times

It is estimated that 85-90% are handled conventionally, are either treated with hormone drugs or through surgery and when this seems not to be working, assisted reproduction comes into question. This is when I will say,

Go look for them,
Don't think it is only them and not you,
They were not them,
Until I became them,
Yes, you could be them,
Meet them
And get to know them.

WHEN IT DAWNED

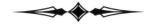

I will never forget this day, 13years ago- I wish I had known what I know today. I lived a quiet and not a rough life, and when I finally settled for pregnancy, I realised it was a battle, a twist of fate for me. When I realised things weren't going on well, having lived for years with my previous partner, I felt need to visit my gynaecologist, I did it initially until the lady doctor insisted carrying out an initial test, which when I came back to her after the dates giving to me, she insisted on seeing my then partner. This took me time to convince him when he did, series of test were carried out, and it was based on the outcome of the test done on him that the initial infertility doctor we met at Uniclinic Dusseldorf recommended IVF treatment.

Invitro Fertilisation (IVF)

Do you know about IVF? He asked us

If you do, that's great. Otherwise, allow me to start this section by explaining what Happens when a couple is going through the IVF process. You can find a lot of information about it in journals and from the hospitals. For the sake of going scientific, my explanation in this book is not conclusive. It is written based on my own experience. It is only aimed at giving an understanding and context, and is not final.

WHAT IS IVF (Invitro Fertilisation)?

Invitro Fertilisation as mentioned earlier, involves hormonally controlling the ovulatory process of removing ovas (eggs) from the ovaries and letting sperm fertilise them outside of the body, in a fluid medium. The fertilised egg (Zygote) is then transferred to the womb so that implantation can occur; cycles are performed each year according to the explanations from one of the fertility doctors.

"You may encounter many defeats, but you must not be defeated. In fact, it may be necessary to encounter the defeats, so you can know who you are, what can rise from you and, how you can still come out of it."

- Maya Angelou.

Yes, like Maya Angelou wrote, defeats encountered helps to know who we are and how strong we are able to deal with challenges. I could say the news looked like a defeat, but in all, it helped me to know who I am.

However, emphasis has been on having a baby and not much on the emotional well-being of couples undergoing this journey. Many women interviewed have described IVF as the most trying period in every couple's life. The truth about this journey is that people are not keen to talk about their failures. Unfortunately, not all IVF is successful, the doctors will tell you too, that does not mean that IVF treatment does not succeed.

This journey requires patience, faith, hope, inner strength and good people around you, because, this particular journey could take you to places that you could never have imagined, and could pose a real challenge that could break or mar you. It took me to places I did not imagine I could go, and it nearly broke me down.

In life, whatever you are going through, have gone through and will go through, always hope to find the right mindset, the strength, the right people and the right voice, to speak out when the time comes, as the time will always come.

After all, I found my voice, and I am going to encourage you through to this journey.

You are special, and you are strong, and you are just unique- you are you, and you are embarking on this journey because you hope to get answers and solutions, so don't stop half way, keep on trying until you excel. The infertility process consumes time, money, energy and saps one's emotion.

"For the bitter experience teaches us a better lesson. Every pain builds us higher strength. Every obstacle leads us to higher ground. The very pain that we felt along our journey is our very best friend. It shall remind us how far we have travelled and how we made it to where we are in the final end."

- Ces Peta.

Yes, this is very true what Ces Peta said about every pain we encounter. This very pain has guided me.

WHERE
YEARNING LEADS

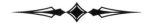

UNIKID DUSSELDORF 2009

At the beginning of this process, we did not have enough money; nonetheless, we needed this joy desperately. With what we saved, and some monetary support from our health insurance we started off(Insurance paid half, and we paid half) this is done for women under 40years, the minute one gets into 40years you are left alone to manage your financial burden. The truth in life is that When you have a need to fulfil, nothing can stand in the way, of your success except you. I guess many who have gone through this journey must have seen themselves in this situation at first.

Yes! the world first stood still and crumbled for a while, as one is told of IVF. You will need at this point a shoulder to cry on, and real-time to digest what was about going to be your own journey or ride.

Initially, there will be this denial that goes with this phase. No, it is not true, it can't be me, why me, and many whys follows until after a while. Seminars and talks on IVF would be suggested for couples, but as at this point, it only depresses, first one would not want to identify oneself with the Terms of infertility. Why, and at the same time, it would be improper not to try.

At this point, try to encourage your partner and assure him. Unfortunately, for a typical African man is shaped and moulded into culture to believe a woman is always at fault.

Most importantly; Do the fight and walk the lane together while treating one another with love, compassion, and understanding this goes a long way to helping the couple deal with IVF journey.

Don't ever walk alone.

 I repeat.

Don't ever dwell on losses.

Do the right thing, ask, and our God and the medical teams will be there for you.

What happens at this stage?

First thing before, loads of papers:

Begins to flow. The doctor will use all the time to clarify every definitions, terms and stages and what to expect.

Clarification over overstimulation of the ovaries due to use of hormonal drugs and the dangers of multiple pregnancies (Aufklärung über Hyperstimulation and Mehrlingsrisiko (Clarifications over the hyperstimulation of the ovaries and the risks of multiple pregnancies with the use of drugs like Menogon, Humegon, Peroganal, Fertinorm, Gonal F, Puregon, Is the German intentional?

With all its implications like Cysts, vomiting, increase in weight, and so forth.

Although, some very lucky ones have been reported with pregnancy during the treatment.

In some cases, depressive reaction has been reported on IVF failures, which can eventually threaten a relationship or couples.

PAPERS TO SIGN:

Consent paper for IVF treatment and the embryo transfer.

Consent paper for general anaesthesia.

Consent for IVF treatment and embryo transfer (einwilligung zur durchführung der IVF und embryo-transfer)

Consent for general Anastasia (aufklärung für IVF/ und vollnarkose)

General consent for other operative matters(einverständniserklärung für allgemeine und operative behandlung.

Clarifications on ICSI (Aufkärung für die Durchführung de Intrazytoplasmastischen Spermiuminjektion (ICSI) neben Maßnahmen der in-vitro-Fertilisation

Clarifications on the conservation, preservation of the extracted good eggs (Über die Kryokonservierung, die Aufbewahrung und die Behandlung von befurcteten Eizellen im Vorkernstadium (Different price from the original fees). (can we translate to English as well? Still leave the German just add English)

Genetische Test (Genetical test)
Loaded with all kinds of information,
Confused on what to decide,

Stuck in the mind,
Lost in wonder,
What is next!

Thoughts like,
Won't I ever?
Heart sink and is low.
And, and…

I used as much time as I wanted, for this time to brood, cry and try to come to terms with this. This was a very important time for me. However, every woman in this state has the right to feel this way; it is not a crime; it is just a part of healing and acceptance. You will be alright, just cling to God. All the way, I cried a secret cry and exhausted my thoughts, but you will never know.

The Show Must Go On.

In spite of all, I was determined to go on with the treatment, yes this did not take away the doubts and the hidden fears that accompany this journey.

"Our doubts are traitors and make us lose the good
we oft might win by fearing to attempt".

- Shakespeare.

Fear robs us, and we only can lose if we give in to fears and refuse to attempt.

All done, the day of operation, two eggs extracted, report from the doctor stating that he was able to get two good eggs, that would be fertilised and injected into the womb (Rückmeldung, es konnten 2 Oozyten asserviert werden. A den gewonnen Oozyten wird in-Vitro Fertilisationsbehandlung (IVF).

After the operation which included punctuation to extract the eggs, we were given a number to call in case any complication.

The fertilisation was performed the next day after carrying out every necessary checks, the usual procedure completed.

In our journey of life, we can't always be looking behind when trying to move forward.

At this stage in life, as it is no longer a doubt of doing IVF, it becomes so clear to couples like us then, the natural way to be pregnant was out of scene, that IVF will be the only option left for to conceive, just no need to look back. As I mentioned before, the show must go on.

Again, and again, the world was Thorned and broken into pieces. Many questions as to why me! kept on filling the mind and the mind began to wonder on where to get answers, and the heart ran the race of its life.

At the dawn of IVF and the initial signings, many couples will go through a number of emotional stress. For many couples, especially the woman, the feeling of the world breaking down follows, the feelings of emptiness anger, frustrations and depression, and worthlessness becomes a part of this journey, as it was then with me.

The truth is that all cases of infertility are not the woman's fault, as I mentioned before. Unfortunately, we live in a truth-denying society, especially those from African background, with its patriarchal hold, a man's world, whereby everything that goes wrong in child-bearing is considered the fault of a woman.

Anyway, this is not the moment for blames or pointing accusing fingers; it is a moment of facing reality and coming to terms with the situation at hand. No one will understand you better, unless one who has gone through this path before, experienced the pain, the shattered hopes and the hopelessness, that is the only person who can tell you what this journey is all about.

So give yourself all the time to realise what is about going to take place in your life, show love instead of bitterness, don't be too hard on your-self or your partner. Pray, seek for strength and look for answers at appropriate places.

Avoid situations and negative people, I repeat; they can be additional stress and not necessarily helpful in starting off this IVF journey.

KEEPING TRACK

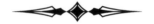

Due to the nature of this journey, the things encountered, like shots taken to stimulate the ovaries, other medications used to assist the egg to mature, preventing of ovulation, timing the medications, Ultrasound, dealing with the financial strains, ups and downs and other things, I started keeping diary on this health journey . I had good and bad memories. Infertility and IVF are such roller coaster, and my way of handing some of the negative feelings and even the good ones was by way of putting some things into writing. Certain things that require step by step, most were noted down. Keeping notes became a way of setting timelines and goals for the journey. With every procedure, every cycle, every call, and how I felt all through, I put in writing. Every stage during the journey cost me a lot of emotional stress, but never deterred me.

Excitement, the unknown, series of test, sweat and tears were words I jotted most on this journey.

"Think about how far you have come today, and how much further you will go tomorrow. You have just to move forward. Each and every step you take must move you towards your goal".

- Dr. -Anil Kumar Sinha.

In all, at every stage, I just have to move forward in thoughts and acts.

This beautiful, painful journey.

A journey of unknown, as painful as it sounds, it is so beautiful and rich in experience.

IVF that great process that involves removing a woman's egg and fertilising it or them outside with sperm in a lab and eventually transferring the embryo back in her womb. As mentioned earlier Eggs removed after hormone therapy, mixed with sperm outside the uterus, after 40 hours, it is expected to be fertilised and take and is placed back into the woman's uterus after ascertaining the thickness of the mucosal lining of the uterus, bypassing the fallopian tubes.

Reportedly, IVF is getting popular since its inception in 1978. It is expensive, involves highly trained professionals, with high technology.

Once these have been ascertained, couple overcoming the initial shock. It is time for the journey to begin; with many consultations, appointments and series of uncomfortable procedures. First consultations, discussions, regarding the hormone treatments, various gynaecological tests till going to a blastocyst stage, and eventually how many embryos to put back.

The first time during this journey follows feelings of relief, because one is getting somewhere and knows that something is being done. When conclusions are made, in whichever cycle to begin, scans are carried out to check the uterine level; this follows next level, stimulation with injections, and tablets. Injections could be painful and hard, because it is not a matter of one shot.

Next will be another scan to check the progress of the ovaries, this is the point that determines increase decrease or end of injection, or if the follicles are not doing well, could lead to the termination of this phase to be started all over again. That's an early shock, must not but could happen.

Most times, all may seem well at the beginning. Going through the normal check and hearing all the time, the good comments from your fertility doctor, makes you think it is all easy. Wait until when things fail to fall in place.

Your world changes the minute anything goes wrong along the journey. Life would not simply look the best, you may opt to quit, but wait, this is too early to make judgement.

This is a very traumatising feeling; you feel alone.

If you have an understanding family, value them, you may not want to share your feelings with anyone at this stage.

Others like Celine Dion and her husband Renee, Lily Becker and some others whom I read their stories on internet, some even reported about having 5-6 failed attempts, as many others shared their concerns their struggles, loneliness, but you may fall into the category of those who lack the courage to do so, because of the feelings that you have failed, and that people will laugh and jeer at you, if you have the choice, don't suffer alone and in silence . Millions of couples are going through this journey, it is not a crime, and you should not be ashamed of yourself.

Don't forget adopting a child is not a crime; surrogacy is also not a crime, modern adoption (use of another person´s egg is not forbidden),be informed and don't kill your dreams of being a mom.

Unfortunately, having all and doing all right doesn't guarantee a safe journey. Sometimes you reflect and think of the many injections of hormones, series of blood tests and scans, this will bruise life and dampen your spirit.

The fear of needles and the thought that what of if?,some of these Questions at every outcome set one into panic, because this is a journey of unknown.

When it fails, you will suffer alone, come back to blames, cry your heart out, and sink into depression, it is true; this is what happens to many in this ride.

The Yearning Journey Continued

"The greatest glory in living lies not in never failing, but in rising every time we fail."

- Nelson Mandela.

As the saying goes when I fall, I rise and fall, I recoil and bounce again.

In each of our visits to any of the reproduction clinics, we were extremely eager, anxious and not knowing what awaits one, but still hopeful and looking forward. Each visit turns out to be different.

I was determined to keep on searching until I found answers. I learnt through prayers not to be afraid to seek new things, and this accompanied me today, even in my profession, I am not afraid of changing workplace and getting into something new.

It was not a first t attempt; at every beginning of this journey, it brings hopes filled with positive expectations. As years pass by hopes, consideration, doubts increases and the question lingers, and the void and emptiness of the mind get worst, because one isn't sure of what awaits one, how many more journeys and if they will ever be successful, or rather, if one will ever be called mom by someone-

Amidst all these, I spoke continuously to God as I tell Him all that was bothering me. I know whatever happens, how long, He will surely hear my cries. I know that God is ever ready to help those who believe and trust in Him.

I thank God all the time, even when I doubt and question Him. He loves me, and takes great delight in my affairs, this I know, because I feel his power in my life. This sustained my fate, increased my strength even when I felt all hopes were lost.

Today, as I recount all, I say to God, God, you have given the doctors knowledge, use these doctors to answer every couple's parental yearnings.

It was in January, when the cold was still on, all arrangement made to start off a journey of another unknown.

It was another attempt, an excellent impression. When the Nurse at the counter with her warm way of welcoming us, ushered us in and there we go.

Mrs, it is your turn. Leaning against the wall, turned and walked into the examination room.

Still thrilled, did not wish any less.

Of course, the question did not depart. Taking out time in between to think, still held my thoughts out, not wanting to think negative, I try to pray each time doubts crosses my mind

Well, upon getting in to the examination room, the soul exclaimed. Had to look up with hope.

My God, I said silently, let it just work this time here in:

Reproductive Clinic Essen

"A difficult situation, is a chance for you and your God", for you to come closer and speak with your maker.

In my whole state, I prayed to God to renew my faith. I cling to him in everything, because I believe in Him because He is loving, caring and will some-day answer me.

Everything in life is a lesson that we can learn from. I remember the first encounter with the gynaecologist, whose radiating smile gave me a real sense of hope. Like in 'Dinner for One' comedy It is just the same procedure, not every day, but every time you go in for this stuff. Having had an encounter before, at least what to expect was not new. Any failure makes us feel grief, and I grieve every time after waiting for 2 weeks only to have a negative pregnancy result.

This is so devasting and crushing; I got crushed many times.

We are in a journey full of routines, when hopes dashes, no short cut, whenever there is change there is loss, and when there is loss there is a grief reaction although no 100% guarantee in any of these cycles, but hope is bound in human existence, and that kept me until losses set in.

"Fall seven times and stand up on the eighth"

-Japanese Proverb-

Yes I failed many times, but my God picked me up each time, and I have a strong faith that kept me going.

Reproductive Clinic in Barcelona.

Having gone through many of IVF attempts that turned out into failures, I began to research again on the internet, hoping to stumble to a site that will answer my yearnings for a child. Yes! All in the journey so far, my faith shrink, still was determined. After a long search, I stumbled into the infertility clinic in Barcelona. I immediately informed my very reluctant partner.

I prayed and asked for divine intervention because that was the only hope I had. At this level of treatment, we had to pay the full cost of the bill, because I was 40years. I saved every money, denied myself a lot and worked double shifts for us to raise another money for another journey. We bought our flight ticket, Ryanair an Irish airline . Having made the contacts on the internet with all the necessary information.

I got my timetable, and after a certain time we were asked for an initial visit to Barcelona for a check and dosage of the hormone, in tablets and injection, and a follow up with my gynaecologist in Germany. This was done faithfully, and both doctors were so happy at the progress of the eggs.

However, the journey of the unknown I called it. The plane landed at a remote Airport, the rest of the information we had to deal with the map which was giving us at the Airport. The next huge problem we faced was language barrier because many we approached for description of the way could not help us, when attempted, they spoke in Spanish.

We continued our search for the clinic, first took a train to a certain place where according to the map, we needed to walk a distance, before we were able to get a Taxi that took us to the clinic.

The good news was that we were being expected, and the ugly news was that we had no hotel close to the clinic, after awhile we got one, a bit far, one of those ordeals peculiar with this journey.

Well, we were there, and all we had to do was to allow divine help from above.

"We should always pray for help, but we should always listen for inspiration and impression to proceed in ways different from those we may have thought of",

- John H. Groberg-

It is so difficult to explain. The healing I know comes from God. I will persist until I succeed, I reassured myself. Always will I take another step. If that is of no avail, I will take another, and yet another. In truth, one step at a time is not too difficult. I know that small attempts, repeated, will complete any undertaking including this difficult journey.

Imagine, making all preparations, getting drained and strained financially, and in the end, not getting that which you have so much sacrificed and hoped for.

My ex-partners sister became a real agony and tormented me in her own ways. Words that came out of her mouth were so negatively powerful that I cried each time and questioned what I was actually doing in a patched relationship, but my hope did not leave me.

Keeping the Hope

That kept me going,
Since I have to go this lane,
walk this walk,
thread these thorns on this journey,
I remembered The Book of wisdom in the Holy Bible
Yahweh created me, first-fruit of His fashioning,
before the oldest of his works.

From everlasting, I was firmly set
The deep was not, when I was born,
nor were the springs with their abounding waters,
before the mountains were settled, before the hills,
I came to birth.

Before he had made the earth, the countryside,
and the first elements of the world,
when he fixed the heavens firm, I was there,
when he drew a circle on the surface of the deep,
when he thickened the clouds above,
when the sources of the deep began to swell,
when he assigned the sea its boundaries.

And the waters will not encroach on the earth,
I was beside the master craftsman,
Delighting him day after day,
Ever at play in his presence,
At play everywhere on his earth,
Delighting to be with (THE PROVERBS 8:22-31).
This gave me a source of hope.

Reproductive Clinic in Cyprus.

With the woes of Barcelona reproductive clinic, my partner and his family lost hopes. His sister pressured him in all forms, but I managed to stay put.

I got information from a close friend who told me about this clinic in Cyprus. I got the telephone number and made the call. Fortunately, they had their visiting doctors in Köln. I immediately made an appointment, and we went for consultations.

I felt the reluctance in him, this nearly discouraged me, but I was yearning and hoping I could get pregnant through IVF wonder.

It was on a Saturday in 2011; we had this appointment where we met 2 Turkey gynaecologists who in their usual calm way, took history, examined me and discussed the necessary cares available. I convinced my then partner, after so many preaching, heartache, He reluctantly succumbed, I borrowed money on my name from the Bank for this journey.

I got in touch with Cyprus, and was in constant touch with AMINA the clinic co-ordinator, a beautiful, soft-spoken lady, who gave us all the assistant we needed, got us a beautiful hotel, arranged for the taxi that came to pick us from the Airport, this was a very good service.

We were picked from the hotel to Nicosia, where the clinic was located. We were treated very nicely for the 14 days we stayed there.

After 14 days of our stay, we had to fly back to Germany, meanwhile, I had a good feeling that it was going to work out.

Behold my visit to my gynaecologist proved me wrong and dashed my world after a negative pregnancy result.

I cried my heart out as I could not understand what was going on again.

This went on and on, until I reached the point where God said to me, enough is enough.

Yes, I cried the cry of cries and blame blames, but could not change anything.

The agony of a woman yearning for a child,
wanting a child badly,
and still could not.

Reproductive Clinic, Nordica-

"Sometimes our light goes out, but is blown again into instant flame by an encounter with another human being."

- Albert Schweitzer.

DOES IVF WORK?

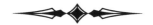

Yes, it does! Well, it did for me, be it after five, six or many failed attempts, it worked the sixth time.

When you have one or two failed journeys, you find yourself grieving. have had to cope even in the face of no hope. I learnt to hold head high above water. in this time, talking can help deal with this process

WHAT I KNOW TODAY

I keep on saying this to me!

All the waiting paid off at God's own time.

"Obstacles don't have to stop you. If you run into a wall, don't turn around and give up. Figure out how to climb it. Go through it, or work around it",

- Michael Jordan-

I encountered a lot on my IVF journey, although, I should give up, but I did not, as I kept on figuring ways of getting to my dream.

Good day and a special day too. Good news is something the soul longs always to have, my very own soul. 16th Nov…..

Our encounter with Nordica changed my whole world positively.

Nov. Good News and a day to remember. The day when the results was what my heart and soul have always longed for. Yes finally, and at last, I got this news that I laboured for so long.

To my Readers - The 'D' Day

Just like the other journey,

When the day of extraction came, the whole procedure done under narcosis, and when you wake up, the tension that follows, asking your-self, "are the eggs healthy"? Because sometimes extraction of eggs does not mean all are ok, the embryologist tells you the number of extracted eggs.

Another journey begins again. You will be told to go home and wait for a confirmation call that will either tell you what next to do or to say sorry, the eggs were unable to fertilise or so… You find yourself waiting and getting panicky at any phone call of any sort. You get agitated, lose appetite and have mood swings. Finally, finally, the call you have been waiting for comes and a voice on the line, that has good or bad news, speaks.

A Crucial Waiting.

This is another crucial stage of your waiting. News that will take you to another level of your journey, news that will shine hopes or dampen your spirit and make you want to quit.

At this moment you don't want to engage in any long talk. All you want to be told, all you want to hear is; "congratulations we were able to fertilise your eggs," or "we are sorry it did not work-followed.

You are expected at the clinic at so and so time, for the transplantation of the embryo, or the other way round.

On This Day

Back to the clinic on the transfer day, I had a mixed feeling, based on my past journey, but kept praying for things to go well. The implantation process lasted about 30 minutes, following which I was told to lie down for another 30 to 60 minutes. In one's own eyes, everything is carried out according to instructions. I followed all the instructions and was exceptionally very careful.

Now, for the first time, the two-day embryo was implanted. There were hopes, fears, and leaps of joy. Some people may decide to take leave, but the embryologist told me to go about my normal life and try to avoid any stress of all kinds.

The uncertainties in the first attempt made me take 15 days leave from work. On the 15th day, the test was carried out to ascertain the success or failure of the IVF.

The nurse said Negative. First, I felt it was not my result, and wanted another test, which she asked me to repeat the next day...

Those were endless waiting's; I felt feels like exploding in my thoughts, my head, I lost my appetite.

The repeated test did not change anything. My hopes were dashed; my heart was broken again.

Journey Number Six

Six months after I recovered from the shock, I went back to my gynaecologist who had time to talk with me. She encouraged me and gave me referral paper that will take me through to another journey. I had been through these processes five times in my previous relationship. You can't imagine the agony, the pain of feeling isolated, of seeing most of my mates, friends and even my junior ones getting easily and naturally pregnant. Of course, the question lingered in my mind. "Why me?"

I made a more thorough search on the internet; asked friends; sought advice, and even went to Spain all on a quest for answers.

Unfortunately, none of the clinics could give me the positive answers I was yearning for, the chance of having a baby, being complete and finally being happy. Despite all these negative answers, I knew deep down me, there was this fighter in me, who was not ready to give in to all these negative results.

I then opted for adoption, which my then partner agreed and later disagreed due to the pressure. Incidentally, the relationship could not stand the pressure, and we broke up. I then suffered the separation and all the pain and sadness that went with it. Another load of pain and sadness was added on top of what I was already carrying.

I was lost. I lost all hopes. I thought my world was ending, and my dreams were shattered. In short, although I gave up the idea of getting married, I never gave up the burning desire to be a mother.

After about six months of suffering from the separation, I ran into my husband in a supermarket, and that was it.

We told our stories; he heard my story and was ready to take another journey with me.

Six months after we met, he proposed marriage, and six months later, we got married legally in court and church. The joy that follows could not be described — God′s own time.

We decided to take another IVF trip, of course at our own cost, because insurance was not going to assist once you are 40 years old and above and I was 45years.

At this time, I was so knowledgeable about the IVF process. I wish what I knew at this time If I had known earlier. I undertook long research; I found an incredible recommendation about a clinic in Nigeria. I received so much support from my family (Da Franca, Da Ange, My nephew Chimeka and my Anti Teresa, my niece Linda, my sister Vivian Timothy, Sister Gloria and my husband, Hagen were all sources of encouragement to me. A year after we were married went through the IVF again.

This time it worked… finally, **I had a positive result**. Thank God, I achieved my goal. Praise the Lord! I must confess that nothing can be exchanged for one's family. I have a family that I am so proud of. Thank you, Family.

Lessons and Advice TO MY READERS

To all those who are intending to embark on this journey and those who have made more trips.

I have had my journeys, and that is why I am taking time to let you know that you are not alone, and will never be alone on this journey. As difficult as it looks, still many have made success from it. In this journey, as difficult as it may look, will advice anyone

To show yourself love instead of bitterness, don't be too hard on yourself or your partner. Pray, seek for your strength and look for answers at the appropriate places. Although one cannot give you a hundred per cent answer or a shortcut to this journey.

Everyone's journey is not the same, be positive and don't be discouraged in your journey.

Avoid situations that are not encouraging, especially negative people; they can be additional stress and not necessarily helpful in starting off this IVF journey.

The IVF journey is not an easy journey, but what journey is easy in life? No matter what, dare to embark on the journey; it is worthwhile. Make it your journey and be patient. Many couples who were interviewed described this journey as one of the most unpredictable, devastating, heart-aching journey ever. But it can be made, with so many positive results along the way.

If you don't try, you will not know what it means to fail.

Don't forget life itself is a risk, and risk is there to be taken. You have to try, and not get scared. After all, you will never know if you don't try. You will realise how much stronger you are in the face of failures; perhaps, one of the most challenging journeys you will ever take in your life. You will learn to never quit in the face of any challenge, and in the end, it will make you very strong.

Of course, I see it as a challenge; for whatever reasons, it was not in God's plans to challenge any couple with this. No woman is born barren and for the fact that you have to go this journey does not make you any different from any other woman.

It may sound hard, but you are different, you may not end with heartbreak. You may be one of the few lucky ones that make it in one trip. Bear this in your mind, in case if you want to take this journey. Go with faith, for, in the end, it is only but the faith that will take you a long way.

IVF is very safe according to medical experts and is nothing to be ashamed of. Once you are left with this option, make sure your doctor explains everything to you and your husband.

Research and inquire after clinics with success rates. Plan your programmes, which include your work, take a holiday. Discuss cost and be very sure. Have an open mind, the journey can be exciting and at the same time nerve breaking.

Be well informed at any stage, ask for every test done on you, and prepare as many questions as possible.

After many trips that failed, one is bound to have luck even if it means once. Most couples have broken up because of the failure of the woman to conceive. Naturally, cases of divorce, bullying of the woman from the partner and even in-laws have been reported.

This is the time people will come up with different accusations. Some may even say oh, she was wayward. Even the man who medically is responsible for this will allow you to be frustrated.

Sometimes and even all the time, most things happen for a reason. Separation may be God´s ways of telling you. My child, I have something better for you. I suffered separation when this journey was not yielding positive results.

After I got separated from my ex-partner, I met my husband, my love, my hope and my God sent. Who took me for what I am and was ready to journey with me?

Good news is good for the body, the whole system. How will it look like when all our days are filled up with good news? The heart is relaxed, the body is at peace, and the system functions well, and the mind finds its peace and work goes on.

What can I say and what can I offer you, my dear Lord?

When I started this journey, the days were as if it would never come to an end. I stopped counting the days and allowed the days to count for me. Jesus is the answer, and Jesus answered me.

On this day, the day that has gone into my good record, a day I have set aside as a special day. The ultimate day that measured where I stand where I should be and where God intended for me. At times of challenge and controversy, it takes a lot of courage.

As they say, tough times never last, but tough people do. This was a journey I started years back, every time I hoped for good news, never did it come until at God´s perfect time.

I have failed over and over again in my life, I did not give up, even when I should have,

I felt lost, almost at the verge of losing touch with reality. My confidence started to shrink, hopes were turning up hopeless, I nearly almost gave up, but God gave me the power to fight even when am failing.

I picked up courage, looked for a solid foundation to rebuild my life again and Jesus was the pillar, my rock and my salvation.

"Making your mark on the world is hard. If it were easy, everybody would do it. But it's not. It takes patience, it takes commitment, and it comes with plenty of failures along the way. The real test is not whether you avoid this failure, because you won't. It's whether you let it harden or shame you into inaction, or whether you learn from it; whether you choose to persevere."

- Barack Obama

Yes, I chose to persevere, and I thank God for our bundle of joy.

CULTURAL VIEWS ON IVF FAILURE.

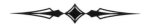

How to deal with the psychological effects of invitro fertilisation.

Sometimes we recall a memory and its associated feelings, but sometimes we experience an old grief feeling without a connected memory and ends up merging with our current grief reaction in healing grieving people when tears are not enough.

It is the sensitivity of our culture and the act of dealing with some unforeseen conflicts between our psycho-social and self that is our greatest challenge in this yearning. The implications are: we think more, react to issues and even tend to recoil and get sad.

We are not only compelled by our personal confrontations worldwide when situations deviate from societal norms; rather we tend to succumb to the demands and thinking of those around us, and allow them to define situations for us.

Pregnancy like any other situation is not only biologically defined, our cultural and religious background, have so far influenced the way and manner in which we define what is natural pregnancy and unnatural pregnancy which "IVF" is viewed and subjected as unnatural.

However, the view of IVF by some groups and culture as not natural remain a sensitive issue that exists in all components of our society.

Closely looking at the nature of the effect of infertility of various tradition, beliefs, religion we see that culture influences through its ways of definitions, pressure on newly married couples.

No wonder, the nature of couple's grief is influenced by so many factors. Many other factors affect couple's reaction. Hence, this book is aimed at helping all see the cultural environment in which we live and thrive, also to extend the importance of respecting people ´s situation especially in IVF failures and infertility cases and in their grieves.

We all grieve, failures are part of our journeys in life, and unfortunately, people I have encountered in the course of this journey, many do not want to talk about IVF, this is seen as a human trait. As an insider and others, we must be aware of cultural and societal effects so as to connect with the grieving and the psychological trauma that goes with this ride.

How do we encourage others to develop their coping concept, at what stage do we accept failure?

We tend to associate grief with loss and failures, but grief can be as a result of other things. References to stories of others show that everyone is different in the way we relate to failures. Most times, grief is associated with loss or death. Other than being sick, losing jobs, divorce and others. IVF failure or infertility could be very depressing and could cause a high degree of grief.

DEALING WITH IVF GRIEF AND PAINS.

We can never deny pains, neither can we pretend that it never exists. We live in a world full of challenges, ups and downs,

A world where we can never have it always our ways. However, one great thing about this book is the expression of pains that goes with IVF and how society threatens the healing process.

Sadly, in most of our African culture, we are forbidden from freely talking about certain things, such as failure to conceive naturally, mental health issue and many more. This is unlike in western culture.

Some ways in which African Culture defines situations can leave you baffled with shock. Culture can make us and at the same time mar us.

What do we even appreciate as culture?

Everything, all, especially for those of us from Africa. This is a crucial aspect of life. We all seek to belong somewhere and our culture, whether good or bad shapes who we are.

Healing Through Listening

"Listening to other people's IVF stories."

This is to suggest that hearing that others have gone through this yearning of seeking for a child, and have come out in the end with success, makes the journey bearable and worth going. Though one way to praise these people is by learning from the strength which in itself reflects courage, persistence and prayers.

Celine Dion and her late husband's Renee´s tale of their IVF journey, Lily Becker, and others are inspiring, as they help through freely talking about their encounters---

This brings back that kind of powerful … feelings that give meaning to life—losing hope, struggle between dreams, and the …. Drawing of strength from personal experience.

The things that concern us most is to be able to deal with our dilemmas. Stories of others are very powerful.

"The greater the difficulty, the more glory in sur-mounting it. Skilful pilots gain their reputation from storms and tempests",

- Epictetus

Life is not all about success; it is also about failures, loss and disappointments. These life´s challenges are certainly things we are bound to encounter in our life´s journey, whichever, it is sure there, and we can't simply avoid it, so be ready to deal with obstacles when they come your ways.

It does not help so much to look constantly at the past; otherwise, you will miss the next train taking you to your future.

Find something positive to occupy you and keep yourself busy, when I was not writing; I engaged myself into one study programme or the other! Books and pens became my companion, my tools and the way of letting out.

I can't tell you that it was an easy journey. Many of you that have walked on this lane may know what I am talking about. It is not all about pains, the desire, the waiting, and the counting of days. It is all about you, and what happens when all efforts were not rewarded? What do you do, cry your heart out, resign or give up hopes?

Many of us have ways of dealing with issues. I dealt with my empty, lonely days through writing. I write and write, because I know there are so many out there itching to hear other people's story. Instead of breaking my head and wondering what went wrong, I learnt to do it this way.

The thought that always goes with each attempt is, oh it would be great if this turn out positive

"Too often, we underestimate the power of a touch, a smile, a kind word, a listening ear, an honest compliment, or the smallest act of caring, all of which have the potential to turn a life around"

-Leo Buscaglia

They were impossible odds that could hold one back from success; I tried to overcome these failures, disappointments, each time I am stricken down, I refused to let the fear of defeat accompany me, of course, I had my moments when I let my emotion just flow.

It was so natural for me those days to worry, to break down and cry; it was something very natural to cry to God and tell Him my stories, despite Him knowing it all.

This is you talking to yourself and learning the way of healing your wounds and encouraging others to learn the best method to face tough situations.

It will encourage you emotionally and equip you to make a successful journey even if it means you taking more than one trip.

Don't forget! Life is hard at times, but when faced with life's challenges, failures, disappointments and deprivations, don't kick against others, be strong, embrace them and seek God's support.

How do we cope with the psychological strains, the stigmas and the pains?

As Robert Schuller said; problems are not a stop signs, they are guidelines. Hope is important because it can make the present moment less difficult to bear. If we believe that tomorrow will be better, we can bear a hardship today.

Learn to do things with calm
Seek those who understand your pains.
Know when you are choked.
Depression is real.
Talk to someone.

Never let your head hang down. Never give up and sit down and grieve. Find another way. And don't pray when it rains if you don't pray when the sun shines IVF one of the most complicated treatment options for infertile couple, a last chance option for a most desired hope does not have a 100% success rate, there is always this fear that accompanies one that even after spending money, doing the right thing, does not guarantee in most cases a successful journey.

When it fails to work, you end up with nothing in your hands to show for all the pains agony and all efforts. This could paralyze one to inactivity; one is emotionally vulnerable, very upset, mentally and frustrated. Talking about it makes the matter worst and unbearable for the woman, especially in some culture that give women only the blames.

There is no success without trials, errors and failures, and there is no success without hard work and sacrifices. See your case as not different from others, millions are suffering like you, and millions will still suffer. Although millions are succeeding too, but whenever, if you are not lucky this time, try again. Nothing is impossible with God.

Pain and anxiety dominated me, ruled me, and, engulfed me. They can leave their mark.

It is worst for the woman than it is for the men. I am not trying to say that men are emotionless, rather men in their nature have learnt to oversimply issues and tend to take it more lightly.

For the woman, there is this social pressure to which infertile couples are subject to. Women suffer more because in most cultures and religion, women are believed to be the infertile ones and not the men. There is nothing you can do to change this notion, even when medical tests prove otherwise, the blame somehow goes to the woman, who the society believe was rough with her sexuality.

Infertility is an extremely emotional experience, affects one's esteem, you feel bad about yourself, if not careful could shake one's faith in God, or in most extreme cases can break marriages. Cases have been reported about the quest for IVF as being all-consuming, crumbling and wrecking.

Price of infertility can be immense, when faced with this think of it as a challenge, learn to overcome this, study cases and sap strength, in the end, the strength you can derive from this battle can be a very healing experience.

Let go of your frustrations, stop blaming yourself, get committed to your efforts and your goals, don't let this negative, sisters-in-law destroy your person, there are likes of them everywhere. Surround yourself with positive people who believe in you.

This journey, when faced with God, supports and carefulness can teach you a lot of lessons, it is up to you to consider which lessons you want to take out of it.

So many women get pregnant every day in a natural way. At this thought, one begins to wonder why me. It is most disturbing when the doctor has done all the test and keep on telling you; there is no problem, everything is ok. Until everything is not taking its natural place.

One feels so sad like the world is emptying on you. What follows is sorrow, hurt, anger, this is very normal, no reason to feel bad about your sad state.

How long and how far with this feeling?

This is a question most couples asked themselves after 2 or 3 attempts. Unfortunately, the number of dropouts after a failed first attempt is usually high, due to cost and stress factors. The next thought is clouded with other available options.

What is the next step?

What other options are available for us?

Querying and searching on the internet for any new information to this topic is considered very important.

Go for whatever makes you happy, your life is precious, and every choice you make could either make or mar you.

Don't take decisions alone, whatever, your partner is the first point of consultations. Learn the way of mutuality; he is your partner.

I spent so much time, years, money, emotion and sleepless night on IVF journey.

Time heals, I am getting there. Not easy though, but it was a choice not to go half way

This journey made me want to question God at some stage. It was so emotionally killing, too much pain that became so hard and made me so hard as a rock.

I did not initially want to identify myself with the reality that I have gone through this journey, it became my story, and I became a part of this journey. It is not a crime if it does not work for you, at first or second attempt.

I refused to talk about this journey for several years, maybe because I was not yet ready, not prepared, or have not find the right time as this time.

Choose your right time to talk about your pains, share with others, because there are a lot out there dying to hear your story.

I needed the courage to talk about this journey, with time, it became easier to talk, deal with and here I am today, writing this book for the world to read and learn. Whether or not you have had to go through this journey. This book will help you understand first hand the experience of a woman yearning for a child. You may relate if you are going through the process, or you may understand and be able to support someone who is going through struggles of having a child.

"Courage doesn't always roar. Sometimes courage is the quiet voice at the end of the day".
I will try again tomorrow",

- Mary Anne Radmacher-

Every life is different, and every journey is different and carries with it its failures and success. But this is our journey. When I look back, I have reasons to thank God. That he kept me alife and gave me the means to keep on fighting until I succeeded.

I had reasons to give up after so many failures; I did not

Many are out there that desperately would want to go along in this journey; they can't because there is no money.

Don't forget failed IVF is not the worst penalty, there are so many other horrible sufferings than this failure so be thankful to God

It hurts I know, nonetheless feel happy for others, share their joys, and don't feel pity for yourself. Care and be pleased for others; caring can bring out the best in you. So, care for others if you can't carry your own. Give love; there is a lot in giving and in loving others.

Don't give yourself up. You will hear talks, and you will inevitably encounter situations that will bring you back to thinking lane.

No one said it is secure. But learn to deal with issues the calm way. It may take years of experience, failures before you realise what I am saying now. When you learn to do this, you see things begin to happen.

When I began this journey years back, I had the eagerness to become a mother like any other woman.

The thought of it, the excitement and the euphoria, carried me on through the journey.

I was naive, despite being told about the plus and minus, I did not indeed realise that anything could fail. I busied myself, concentrating on being a mom.

I can't tell you how many injections, and pills that I took.

The two weeks of taking injections, swallowing drugs, meeting appointment until the day the specialists okay the eggs and the number.

At the first attempt, I wasn't nervous, because there was this belief sustaining me.

The outcome of any IVF journey is always uncertain, the only practical way is to move forward by taking action, and when it fails take more action, whatever that action is to you. Some people give up; others keep fighting. There are many factors at play when you are in this situation, and there is no 'one size fits all' answer. Every woman is different. Go with your gut instinct and even your financial situation, unfortunately.

Do it, follow the process, take as much journey as you can afford so that in the end you will look back with the thought, I did my best.

In the next chapter, I will share my experience of looking after myself mentally and physically.

MENTAL HEALTH AND WELLBEING

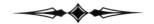

Recognising Your Anxiety.

Situations like repeated IVF failure may contribute to the psychological breakdown of a healthy individual. No one can tell you the best way to prevent or avoid it. Hence, the use of resources around you may be beneficial.

Anxiety state is a neurotic kind of illness of which depressive state is included, and is very common with yearning for a child.

You know your problem, and on the other hand, you can't deal with the confrontations. These are issues arising from unresolved situations like IVF failures.

The body has a way of reacting to psychological stress and feelings that are not normal in our system; these are individually displayed.

Don't forget, depression is real and can occur in association with the failures and journey of IVF. Hence, I advice you to look out for these symptoms. If your low feelings persist, please speak to your doctor.

DEPRESSION the NHS information website (NHS Depression, 2019) is a situation with extreme slowness of movement and thought instead of overactivity and elation. One looks unhappy and complains of misery, guilt lack of interest, low esteem and others.

In worst cases some people have suffered hysteria, leading to self-centred behaviours, with some physical symptoms and some functional abnormalities, these you would be told in the process.

One can also experience frustration, crying, lack of interest in everything, and see only negative side of things. Some of these reactions have broken marriages.

At this stage, don't entertain too much sympathy. You need someone who understands you. But in the extreme case seek out for a psychotherapist, never mind what people would think. You need help.

Psychosis is rear in this case, but could if not managed well, but am not sure it could be too extreme, except those who are predisposed.

On a general note, when you feel symptoms like intense fear, sleeplessness, loss of appetite, don't wait for so long, seek for help, before it gets so bad.

THE LESSON I LEARNED FROM EVERY STAGE OF THIS JOURNEY.

THE D_DAY; The day of extraction came. The whole procedure was done under narcosis and when I woke up, the tension that follows, asking myself questions such as;

Are there any healthy eggs?

Is this going to work this time?

Because sometimes when the eggs are extracted, does not mean all are ok, the embryologist tells you the number of retrieved eggs.

The journey begins, you will be told to go home and wait for a confirmation call that will either tell you what next to do or to say sorry, they eggs were unable to fertilise or so …

You find yourself waiting and getting panicky at any ring of any sort.

You get agitated, lose appetite and mood swings. Finally, the call you have been waiting for came and a voice on the line, that has good or bad news, speaks. This is another crucial stage of your waiting. The story that will take you to another level of your

journey, news that will shine hopes or dampen your spirit and make you want to quit.

At this moment you don't want to engage in any long talk, all you want to be told /all you want to hear is _ congratulations we were able to fertilise ---all you wanted to know at this point was, not how many, the number you find out when you have calmed your joy down.

It follows, Mrs--- you are expected at the clinic at so and so time, for the implantation.

On the Day

Be calm. Do the right thing, be yourself and believe and put your trust in God. Avoid stress, and what negative thing that goes around you. Learn to relax, when you feel like exploding in your thought, don't jump into anxiety, be calm and pray, pray and keep on praying, because the next stage you are about to get in after implantation demands every good luck on earth.

Look unto your partner, sap courage from him. Pray to have a loving and supporting partner who is willing to go through the journey with you, I was so inpatient before, but this journey made me learn how to be patient.

Don't be stressful, fill your mind with prayers, don't upset your system, because worries have never been known to solve any problem, the delayed progress.

Do what makes you happy, when you are delighted, hormone shoot out in your system, everything come into shape, and you are ready to face the next path.

Being calm is better than being hectic. It is difficult sometimes to maintain calmness. Still, you will need to practice it. When you are composing your energy revitalise, you have self-confidence, and you are ready to plunge into the next step.

Lesson I Learnt After Egg Transfer

"Don't forget life isn't worth living unless it is lived for someone else."

- Albert Einstein-

I can only advice you to be optimistic even at this point in your journey. Have a positive mindset, do your best, and leave the rest for God to fix.

No one has a unique talent to cope during this period, but God's will is the best. Pray for confidence and believe in what God can do; this is very important to success. If you don't have the strength, energy and courage, to believe in yourself, continue disturbing God, continue at every given opportunity, pray and pray, until you have it, and continue even after you have it.

Be unique in your thinking, because you're different from the other person. It did not work for A at first attempt does not mean that it will not work for you. We all are different.

Transferring does not mean a 100% success, to most who have gone through this lane 2 or more times know where I am coming from.

This is the beginning of another milestone, as heavy as the thoughts were, I started to carry away the small stones that were to block my thoughts, because this time, I needed to be calm.

This is a long two weeks of waiting after embryo transfer, when I mean long waiting. It is not just like any ordinary waiting. It is a waiting that could mean the world.

Worst of all, it becomes so nervously chilling when you may have done it more than three times as it was with my case. There were moments I had thought of doubts as it creeps into the mind now and then.

You may not even know what to think and would only hope and wish someone tell you the result is positive.

This is a battle fought within your four walls, within you and with you alone., yes! I fought this battle within me, but God was always there in my company.

"Even if happiness forgets you a little bit, never completely forget about it",,

- Jacques Prevert-

Yes, I forgot to be happy, no matter how hard I tried then,

Honestly, I dreaded this moment, because I did not know what was coming.

Like any other person in this journey I hoped for answers, positive answers at each journey the answer every person on this journey hates to hear, is of course, No.

Well, it is not only about the emotion, the expectations that never came, the money borrowed, where do I start, who do I tell these stories and who will understand my agony, if not only me and my God.

The worst of it all is that the world is not standing still because you are sad. Let me tell you. It is not that I m so strong, it is just that I have stayed with problems of IVF for so long . I have no exceptional talent and have no particular skill, I learnt to master the skill, because out of many failures I learnt to fight my way to succeed, to deal with rollercoaster feelings that go with it and to appreciate and respect those in this journey.

I learnt to accept failure as being a part of me and a part of life. This made me keen to challenge myself further as I realised that I was doing something and the same goes to you.

Most times, we allow the fear of failing or losing becomes more significant than the joy of us winning, and we want to give in to doubts, doubts that puts a stop to one's efforts.

Don't choose the way of fears, try once more, or even many times, if it fails to work out, it does not mean that you were never meant to succeed, will urge you to Keep on trying as long as you want to achieve, until you get there,

Try, sooner or later, those who win are those who have accepted the challenges of failure and have learnt to try one more time "-Jeff G. Yes I tried this many times, and I succeeded with the help of God in the end.

When you are down, you are not finished, because God is not finished with you, why should you then give yourself up, when God is there to help?

"man is fond of counting his troubles, but he does not count his joys. If he counted them up, as he ought to, he would see that every lot has enough happiness provided for it",- Fyodor Dostoevsky-

This is very true but was far from me during these failures.

Anything that delays you from achieving whatever plans you set for yourself doesn't mean you should get too angry. Think back and let the truth of the 18th century spiritual writer Jean – Pierre de Caussade sink in ---- "Whatever happens to you in the course of a day, a month, a year, for good or bad, is an expression of God's will, "Instead of cursing your luck, banging your head, or rolling your eyes in frustrations, see the wait, the disappointment as a spiritual invitation - Bishop . Cry and mourn, and don't languish in your pains and don't dwell too much on what failed to be. Shut the world out sometimes and live in your world. Clear your mind and seek God's grace, most importantly don't forget- you have not failed until you have quit "- Guardian B. Hinckley- you are not born to quit, I did not quit, so you will not.

IVF failure is not a one-time success treatment for many when it fails to work at the first attempt be prepared for more journey, don't be ashamed about it. It is not the end of the world.

When the journey fail at any attempt, as it does not promise a 100% success rate, when this journey you are riding seems all rough, when the funds are low, and the debts are high and you think still you are not succeeding, pray, when the thought of this pressing you down as it would, seek God, but do not quit your dream, because you never can tell how close you are to realising your dream .

So stick to God, to your hopes, to your dream, to your fight when you're hardest hit – is when things go wrong that you must not quit" – Author unknown.

So do not quit–

This is my story, and I hope you will benefit and be active even when you think you are not making any progress, learn to believe in God in you and trust what the lord can do in your life. I trusted Him, and I know he was not going to let me down.

I learnt that "when you get into a tight place, and everything goes against you, till it seems as though you could not hang on a minute longer, never give up then, for that is just the place and time that the will turn" - Harriet Becher Stone -

Watch out for my upcoming books, tells the story of persistence that led to success. God answered me. He will also visit you at His right time.

Some friends touch your heart in a way that you can never erase.

ACKNOWLEDGEMENT

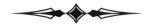

We get to a stage in life when we look back and say oh! Our difficulties and disappointments weren't so bad after all, as long as we do not brood so long on them. Today, I continuously say big thank you to God for using my past failures to make me a better person. I have struggled to discover me through a great gift from God in my husband, Hagen, our bundle of joy, my parents in law Christa and Alfred Meierdierks for being an excellent support for me.

I want to thank my God, my family Umu late Mr and Mrs Patrick Uzodinma Uwazie, and all friends and well-wishers for truly supporting me all through.

I appreciate my older sisters; Adanne Franchesca Uche, Mrs Angela Ndukwu and Pau Pau.

Thank you my other siblings; De Cos, art unleashed Vivian Timothy, my childhood best sister whose artwork has added to the meaning of this book,Bolaji Aina my secondary school bestie, Rev. Sister Gloria Ibe, Rev. Sr Bernett Uduhirinwa, Rev Sr, Chalice Idika, Chinwe. My dearest Ugochi, Chimeka, Amarachi, Ikechi, Nneka, Chinyere Anti Theresa Nwogu, Anti Caro Osuagwu, Anti Mary Jane, and many others not mentioned here. Mr and Mrs Madu and family, Mr and Mrs Chibuike Nwachukwu and family, they stood behind me in this journey.

A big thank you to my publishing company in the UK; Amina Chitembo and her team for their hard work in bringing this book to life and for believing in me.

A big thank you to the Staff of Nordica in Nigeria for helping me realise my yearning for a child.

I would also like to acknowledge the couples that shared some of their pains with me, some staff I met in the process of my journey, May God bless all.

Thanks to Dr Melpani whose on-line teachings on IVF have being so encouraging.

Thanks to Celine Dion and her late husband for being an inspiration through sharing their stories online.

And to you, my readers, friends and fans, thank you for taking time to read this book.

REFERENCES

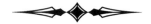

American Pregnancy Association. (2019). Female Infertility. Retrieved July 25, 2019, from APA website: https://americanpregnancy.org/infertility/female-infertility/

Chopin, K. (1984). *The Awakwning* . Penguin Classics; 1 edition.

HFEA. (2019). In vitro fertilisation (IVF). Retrieved July 25, 2019, from https://www.hfea.gov.uk/treatments/explore-all-treatments/in-vitro-fertilisation-ivf/

Mastenbroek, S., van der Veen, F., Aflatoonian, A., Shapiro, B., Bossuyt, P., & Repping, S. (2011). Embryo selection in IVF. *Human Reproduction*, *26*(5), 964–966. https://doi. org/10.1093/humrep/der050

NHS. (2019). Infertility. Retrieved July 25, 2019, from Website website: https://www.nhs. uk/conditions/infertility/

NHS. (2019). Depression. Retrieved July 25, 2019, from Website website: https://www.nhs. uk/conditions/clinical-depression/

Pearce, E. C. (1980). *A General Textbook of Nursing*. Mosby.

Rooij, H. M. (2009, JUly). *Journal of Psychosomatic Obstetrics & Gynecology, volume 28*, 65-68. Retrieved from www.tandfonline.com

UK, N. (2019, July 26). *NHS*. Retrieved from NHS: https://www.nhs.uk/conditions/ infertility/

ABOUT THE AUTHOR

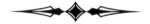

My name is Clara Meierdierks (née Uwazie). I was born in Nnarambia Ahiara, Mbaise, Nigeria, to the late Mrs Elizabeth Adanma Nneoha Uwazie and the late Mr Patrick Uzodinma Uwazie. My mother gave birth to eight children in total.

I am qualified as a Nurse/Midwife, a Quality Manager (Cert.) and have a B.Sc. (Hons) In Health and Social Welfare and an M.Sc. in Psychology. I am also a Respiratory Care Practitioner, as well as being a speaker, a blogger and an author. I am just so happy that I have recently discovered my identity. Yes! Being an author has added so much more colour into my life. I am thankful to God, and to those who have supported me all through.

At the moment I am working with semi-coma and coma patients utilising life support aids, and I must confess that working with such patients has helped to reshape my life in a very positive way. These experiences have brought me closer to the realities of life.

I am very active in the field of women's organisations and empowerment. I am a founder member of CWO Bremen and a member of the CWO at a national level. I am also an active member of 'African Week', an event which is held every year in Augsburg and where I have had the opportunity to speak on the causes of people having to take flight and immigration causes, pains of immigration and their possible solutions. My thanks go to my sister Adanne Francesca, Da Ange, Vivian, Margret Aulbach, Julia Kupa and lots of others who have helped me in these matters.

I love reading and writing. I also love seeing people happy, and I have learnt in the course of my journey to master patient, I believe in forgiveness and pray that those I may have offended should forgive me. I do not hold anything against anyone, because it is a burden to do so, and I love my peace.

I believe that we all are born to be creative and the world is big enough to contend all our talents and stop us from competing with one another, no matter where we find ourselves, or the challenges we go through in life. We should not leave God behind, for through prayers, we get our strength and faith, and through faith and hard work, the sky will be our starting point.

Just like any other person, I have gone through many challenges and have fallen many times. I believe in never quitting - fight, pray, pursue your dreams, and the universe will do the rest.

PRAISE
FOR THE BOOK

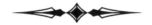

I have taken time to read these inspiring words. I had an IVF at one attempt, and due to the pains and the loss I suffered after a failed attempt, I immediately opted for adoption.

This is a book filled with emotion, a true journey. All I can say is thank you, Clara, for being bold to talk about this topic. As an African, I know what it means, and that is why, I will urge all out there to please buy this book, support this author.

She is doing great work in using her story to empower many out there. I could go on to sing praises on this book.

Once more, thank you, Clara. If I had known this, I would not have stopped halfway, but thank God; I am happy with my beautiful children.

Please, as the author wrote, don't shy away from your problem, Infertility is real, IVF is real, depression is also real, and the good news is that you don't have to die without being a mom, you can adopt, there is surrogacy I know many countries allows that. If you have the money, try IVF when natural ways fail.

Every woman is a good mom, be a mom to someone, all you need do just be a good mom, in the end, no one cares if you're the biological mom or not, all that matters is you being good.

Thank you.

MARY JANE

COVER ART

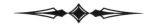

Dr. Vivian Timothy- Art Unleashed
Name: *Self-Evolution.*
Acrylic on Canvas 60/80cm.
Website: *www. art-anleashed.com*

Description: Prose

Self-Evolution
 Painting Myself Out of My Cage,
Liberating Myself From my fears and doubts,

Please! Don't tell me I have arrived,
I am still on my journey to self,
Breaking free from the shackles of my past with
my Brush and colours.

Evolving as a person,
Still evolving,
Keep evolving.

FINAL REMARKS

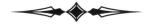

Firstly, thank you for taking time to read my book. Your reviews are important to me. So here is my request. If you enjoyed this book and learned something from it, you can help me in one or more of the following ways:

→ Go online, my website www.claram.net, or on www.amazon.de (or Amazon in your country), then write a kind review. I will greatly appreciate your support, and other readers will be encouraged to read my work

→ Let us connect on LinkedIn: https://www.linkedin.com/in/clara-meierdierks-606001164/.

→ Attend one of my trainings or seminars

→ Email me if I can be of any help with your training or awareness raising events at claram@claram.net. I do reply directly.

→ Get a copy of this book as a gift to your friend or family.

→ Continue to grow to the next level of your life and build the happy life and success you want.

THANK YOU.

BOOKS BY CLARA

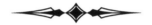

Clara is a prolific writer, has written and co-authored a number of books including the following books also published by Diverse Cultures Publishing. You can find the full collection of Clara's books on Amazon in your country or on her website www.claram.net

Solo Books

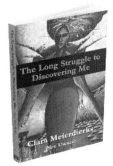

The Long Struggle to Discovering Me
Published: 21 Nov. 2018
Paperback: 144 pages
Publisher: Diverse Cultures Publishing
Language: English
ISBN-13: 978-0995739611

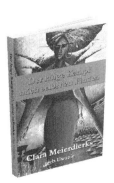

Der lange Kampf mich selbst zu Fin-den
Published: 6 Jan. 2019
Paperback: 162 pages
Publisher: Diverse Cultures Publishing
Language: German
ISBN-13: 978-1916011403

Coming Out in May 2019

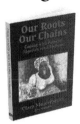

Our Root Our Chains:
Coping with the Nigerian Elections.
Published: May 2019
Language: English
ISBN: 978-1-9160114-4-1

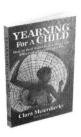

YEARNING For A CHILD: How to Deal with the Psychological Effects of Infertility and IVF. (This book)
Language: English
ISBN: 978-1-9160114-2-7

Co-Authored Books

Clara has contributed chapters in books including these books

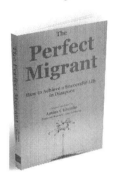

The Perfect Migrant: How to Achieve a Successful Life in Diaspora.
Paperback: 224 pages
Publisher: Diverse Cultures Publishing (27 May 2018)
Language: English
ISBN-10: 0995739692
ISBN-13: 978-0995739697

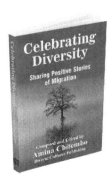

Celebrating Diversity: Sharing Positive of Migration
Paperback: 220 pages
Publisher: Diverse Cultures Publishing (17 Oct. 2018)
Language: English
ISBN-10: 0995739684
ISBN-13: 978-0995739680

Visit Clara's Website to Learn More and check out the latest releases at:

www.claram.net

26009645R00090

Printed in Great Britain
by Amazon